Daily Routine for a

HEALTHY LIFESTYLE

Welcome Message

Welcome! I'm thrilled that you've decided to take the first step toward living a healthier, more balanced life. This eBook is designed for anyone looking to build healthier habits, whether you're just starting or have been on this journey for a while. Think of this as your personal guide to a daily routine that nurtures your body, mind, and spirit. Let's work together to create lasting changes that will leave you feeling more energized, focused, and in control of your well-being.

Table of Contents

INTRODUCTION.

Importance of Establishing a Daily Routine

Life can be busy and overwhelming, but having a daily routine helps you take control.

Establishing a routine simplifies your day, making it easier to accomplish tasks and take care of your health. When you follow a consistent plan, your body and mind adapt to healthy patterns, which helps reduce stress and improve your overall well-being. Daily routines give you structure, help you avoid unhealthy choices, and allow you to manage your time better. Most importantly, small habits practiced regularly can lead to lasting and meaningful improvements in your health and happiness.

A routine also helps with maintaining balance. By dedicating time to self-care, fitness, and healthy eating, you're giving yourself the opportunity to thrive, even on your busiest days.

Whether it's making time for breakfast, taking a short walk, or practicing mindfulness, these small actions build up to create significant positive effects in your life.

Overview of What the eBook Covers

This eBook is your step-by-step guide to building a healthy daily routine that fits into your lifestyle. You'll find actionable tips and advice for each part of your day, from morning routines that set the tone, to afternoon practices that keep you energized, to evening habits that help you wind down and prepare for restful sleep. We'll cover the importance of balanced meals, staying active, and incorporating mindfulness into your day. Each section will break down easy, practical step you can take to stay healthy, energized, and mentally focused.

Whether it's finding time for exercise, making nutritious meals, or practicing relaxation techniques, this eBook is packed with simple, realistic strategies that you can implement at your own pace. The aim is to help you create a routine that not only improves your physical health but also supports your mental well-being. By the end, you'll have a personalized routine that works for you, no matter how busy life gets. Let's get started on creating your healthiest and happiest self!

Chapter 1: Morning Routine

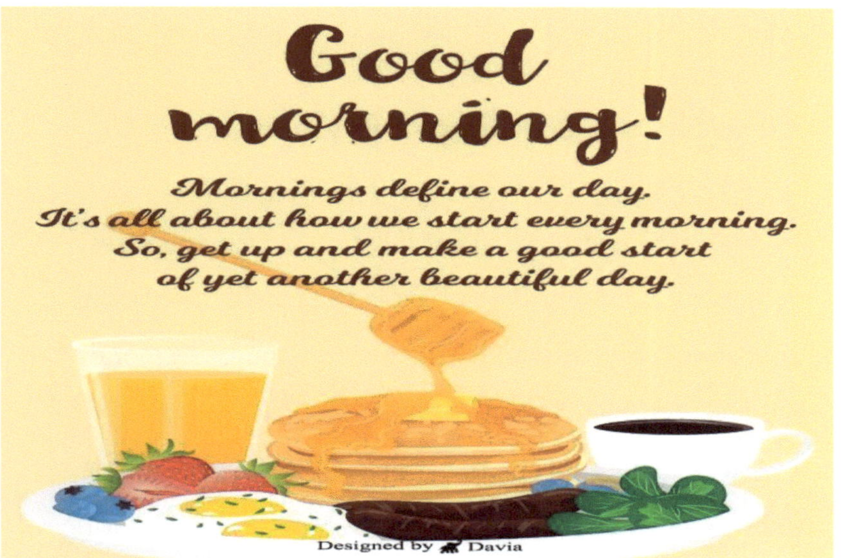

Wake Up Early

Setting the Tone for the Day: Waking up early gives you the gift of quiet, uninterrupted time for self-reflection and planning. This peaceful space lets you gather your thoughts and envision your goals for the day. Start with deep breathing to clear your mind, then think about the actions you want to take and the positive outcomes you want to manifest. This mental alignment sets the stage for a more productive and purposeful day. Consider writing your thoughts in a journal, affirming your intentions to stay on track.

Hydration and Stretching

Energy Boost: After hours of sleep, your body is dehydrated and stiff. Begin by drinking a full glass of water to rehydrate and stimulate circulation, which energizes your mind and body. Stretching in the morning wakes up your muscles, promotes flexibility, and enhances blood flow. Whether it's a gentle stretch or a few rounds of morning yoga or tai chi, this practice brings calm and physical vitality to your start. It also helps release tension from your body, setting a stress-free tone for the day ahead.

Mindfulness Practices

Setting Intentions: Incorporate mindfulness practices to cultivate a peaceful mindset. Breathing exercises, like deep belly breaths or alternate nostril breathing, help calm the nervous system and ground you in the present moment. Following this, set clear, intentional goals for your day. Consider asking yourself, "What kind of energy do I want to bring to today's tasks?" and "How do I want to feel by the end of the day?" By answering these questions, you'll approach your day with clarity and intention, making challenges more manageable.

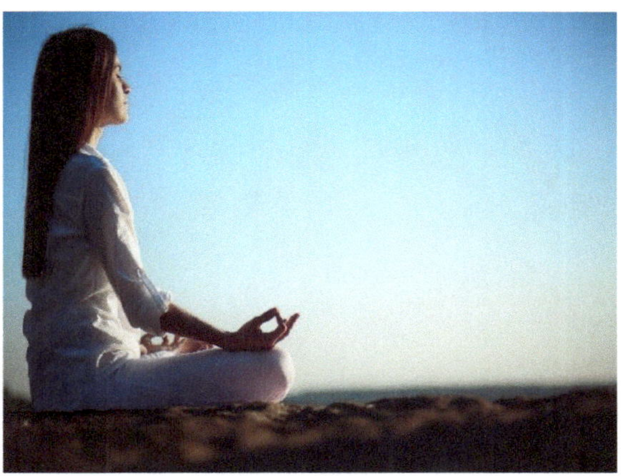

Healthy Breakfast Choices

Fueling Your Brain: A nutritious breakfast is crucial for cognitive function and sustained energy. Choose foods rich in vitamins, minerals, and healthy fats. Chia seeds, oats, flaxseeds, and berries are excellent superfoods that boost brainpower and focus. For a balanced meal, include a source of protein, healthy fats, and fiber to keep you full and energized. A smoothie with spinach, banana, almond milk, and chia seeds is a quick option. This healthy start nourishes both body and mind, setting you up for an efficient and focused day.

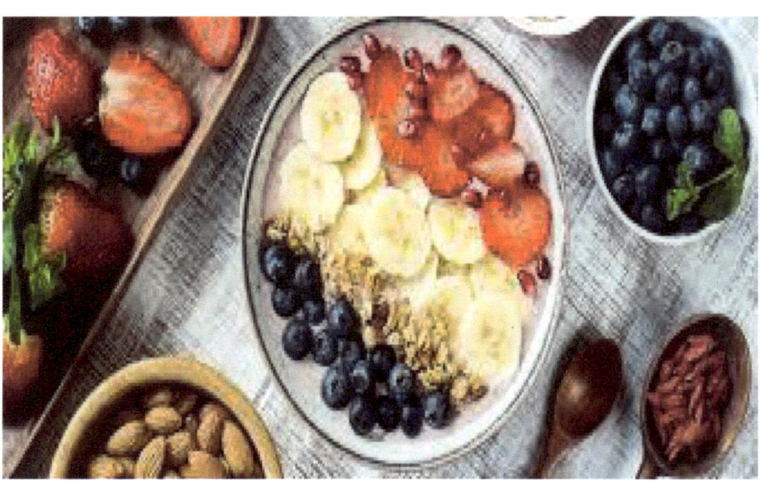

Chapter 2: Mid-Morning Practices

Short Movement Breaks

- **Staying Energized**: Even standing up for a few minutes can boost circulation and get oxygen flowing to your brain. Consider doing a couple of squats, a brisk walk around the office or house, or some quick arm stretches to feel rejuvenated.

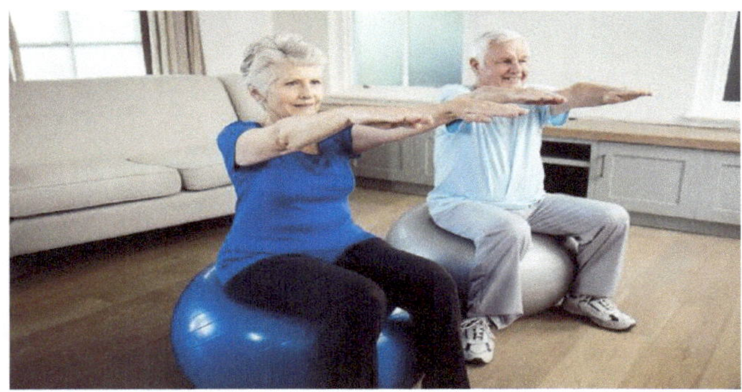

Healthy Snack Options

- **Mindful Eating**: Chew slowly and savor your snack. This mindful approach to eating prevents overindulgence and helps you appreciate the flavors and nutrients. It also encourages mindfulness in other areas of your day.

Mindful Productivity

- **Focus on Quality over Quantity**: It's easy to get caught up in crossing things off a to-do list. But focusing on high-priority tasks and giving each your full attention leads to better outcomes and less stress.

Chapter 3: Lunchtime Routine

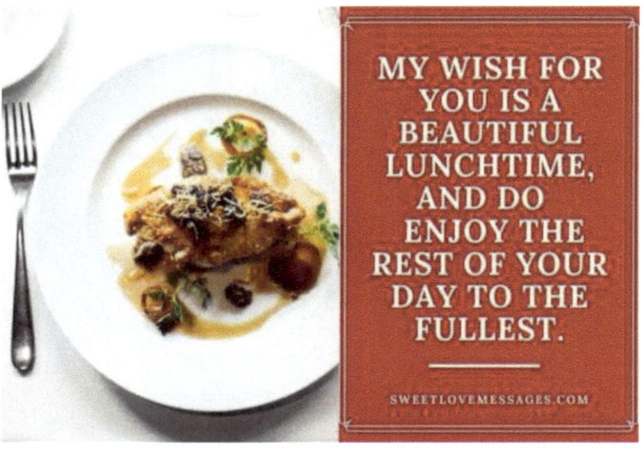

Balanced Midday Meal

- **Supercharge with Superfoods**: Add a variety of colors to your plate. For instance, leafy greens, brightly colored veggies, or a handful of nuts or seeds can give you the necessary nutrients for sustained energy. These foods improve digestion, boost mood, and keep you sharp for the rest of the day.

Avoiding Post-Lunch Slumps

- **Power Naps**: If your schedule allows, a 10-20 minute power nap can refresh you and significantly improve afternoon productivity. Even a short rest can enhance memory, creativity, and focus.

Brief Walk or Light Exercise

- **Mind-Body Reconnection**: Walking helps break up long sitting periods and re-connects you with your body. Use this time for mindful walking, paying attention to your surroundings, the rhythm of your breath, or simply enjoying the fresh air.

Chapter 4: Afternoon Practices

Maintaining Focus

- ☐ **Break down Large Tasks**: Instead of tackling a huge task all at once, break it into smaller, more manageable parts. Crossing off even small tasks creates momentum and keeps you motivated, while reducing overwhelm.

Hydration Check

- ☐ **Infuse Water with Natural Flavors**: Staying hydrated doesn't have to be boring. Infuse your water with slices of cucumber, mint, or lemon to make drinking water more enjoyable. Proper hydration improves cognitive function and prevents afternoon fatigue.

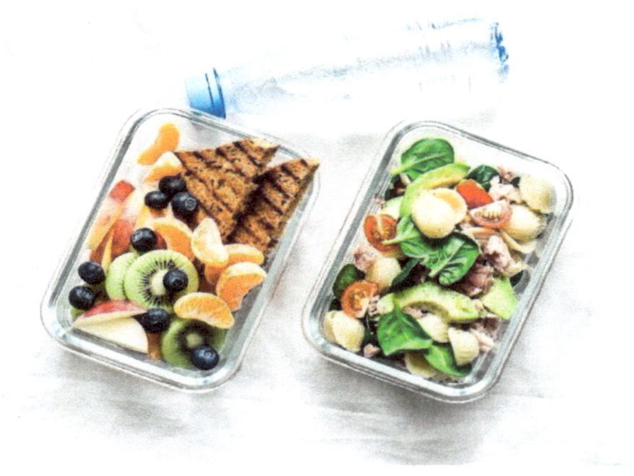

Healthy Snack Alternatives

- ☐ **Energy Sustaining Snacks**: Consider a protein shake, homemade granola bars, or even trail mix with dark chocolate. These snacks provide a balance of fats, protein, and fiber to keep energy levels stable until dinner.

Chapter 5: Evening Routine

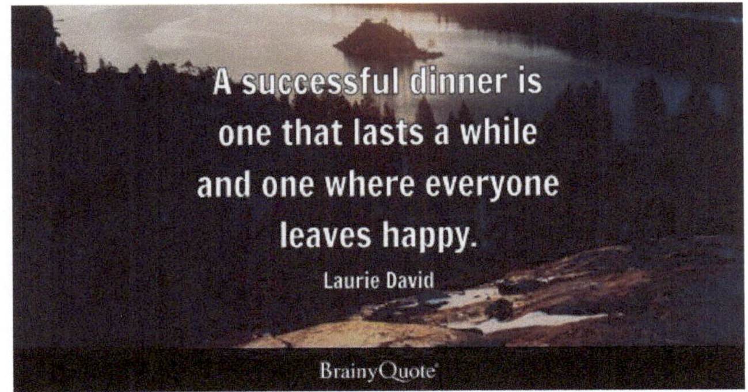

Wind-Down Exercises

Tension Release: After the day's stress, your body might feel tight or fatigued. Engage in restorative yoga poses like child's pose, legs-up-the-wall, or gentle spinal twists to release built-up tension in muscles. Pairing this with controlled deep breathing can lower cortisol levels and improve circulation, preparing your body for rest. You can also try progressive muscle relaxation, tensing and releasing each muscle group, to further relax your body and ease into sleep.

Mind-Body Connection: Take a moment to listen to your body during these stretches. Notice any areas of tightness or discomfort, and allow your body to soften and release with each exhale. Focus on your breath, bringing awareness to the physical sensations. This practice not only helps reduce physical tension but also grounds your mind, shifting your attention away from the day's stresses.

Healthy, Light Dinner

Mindful Nutrient Choices: Dinner should be light but nourishing. Opt for lean proteins like grilled chicken or tofu, and pair them with fiber-rich vegetables like sweet potatoes, spinach, or zucchini. These nutrient-dense options keep your body satiated while aiding digestion and sleep. Try incorporating foods rich in tryptophan, like turkey or nuts, as they can help in melatonin production, promoting better sleep. Avoid spicy or overly acidic foods, as they can lead to indigestion or disrupt sleep quality.

Eat Slowly, Savor More: Pay attention to the process of eating. Focus on the texture, flavor, and aroma of your food, and chew slowly to aid digestion. Eating mindfully allows your brain to register fullness, preventing overeating and late-night snacking. By savoring your dinner, you'll feel more satisfied and emotionally balanced.

Mindful Reflection or Journaling

Daily Reflection: Take time to reflect on your day, either by journaling or mentally reviewing key moments. Consider asking yourself, "What went well today?" or "How did I handle challenges?" By reflecting, you gain insights into your habits and thought patterns, allowing you to approach the next day with greater intention. If you faced difficulties, acknowledge them but also consider the lessons learned.

Gratitude and Affirmations: Journaling about things you're grateful for can have a lasting positive effect on your mental health. Writing down three things that made you smile or feel thankful encourages a mindset of abundance rather than scarcity. You can also pair this with writing affirmations or setting intentions for the following day. This positive self-talk helps shift your mindset, reducing anxiety and enhancing emotional well-being.

Evening Relaxation Ritual

Calming the Mind: The evening is the perfect time to create a ritual that signals your mind it's time to rest. Engage in calming activities like reading a book, listening to relaxing music, or doing light meditation. Choose something that doesn't overstimulate the mind, as this will help transition you into sleep mode. Meditation apps, like Calm or Headspace, offer short, guided sessions perfect for unwinding.

Creating a Sleep-Friendly Environment: Dim the lights in your home an hour before bed to mimic the natural sunset, which signals to your brain that it's time to wind down. Turn off bright overhead lights, and instead, use soft, warm lighting like bedside lamps or candles. Your bedroom should feel like a sleep sanctuary—quiet, cool, and clutter-free. Consider aromatherapy with essential oils such as lavender or chamomile, which can naturally calm the mind and help you drift off to sleep peacefully.

Chapter 6: Night Routine

Digital Detox

Breaking the Screen Addiction: As tempting as it may be to scroll through social media or watch TV in bed, these activities can disrupt your body's natural ability to wind down. The blue light emitted from screens inhibits melatonin production, the hormone responsible for sleep. To create an environment that promotes rest, consider installing an app blocker or setting your phone to "Do Not Disturb" mode a few hours before bed. Establish a "tech-free zone" in your bedroom to prevent distractions and ensure better sleep hygiene.

Relaxation Techniques

Create a Relaxation Ritual: Your brain needs clear signals that it's time to relax and prepare for sleep. Establish a soothing pre-sleep routine that might include lighting calming candles, diffusing lavender essential oil, or playing soft, tranquil music. Incorporating meditation or deep breathing exercises before bed can help release any built-up tension from the day, bringing both mental and physical calmness. You can also practice progressive muscle relaxation, where you tense and release different muscle groups to help your body unwind.

Consistent Sleep Schedule

The Power of Routine: A regular sleep schedule is vital for quality rest. Going to bed and waking up at the same time every day helps regulate your body's internal clock, also known as the circadian rhythm. Build a bedtime routine that signals your body it's time to wind down, such as dimming the lights an hour before sleep, reading a calming book, or enjoying a warm bath. Repeatedly practicing these rituals teaches your body to recognize when it's time to relax, making it easier to fall asleep and stay asleep throughout the night.

Journaling and Reflection

Clear Your Mind: Before going to bed, take a few minutes to write in a journal. Reflect on the day, express gratitude, or jot down anything that's weighing on your mind. This practice helps to clear mental clutter and allows you to go to sleep with a more peaceful mind. Writing down thoughts or to-dos for the next day can help alleviate anxiety, ensuring that you don't lie awake stressing about what's to come.

Creating a Sleep-Inducing Environment

Set the Scene for Sleep: Your bedroom environment plays a crucial role in the quality of your sleep. Ensure that your space is cool, dark, and quiet. Invest in blackout curtains, white noise machines, or comfortable pillows and bedding that promote restful sleep. Consider using aromatherapy to set the mood— scents like lavender and chamomile are known to promote relaxation. A clutter-free and serene room can signal your brain that it's time to rest.

Mindful Evening Snack

Eating for Better Sleep: If you need a snack before bed, opt for foods that promote sleep, such as a small serving of almonds, a banana, or a glass of warm milk. These foods contain melatonin or magnesium, which support healthy sleep cycles. Avoid heavy, spicy, or overly rich foods, as these can disrupt your digestion and make it harder to sleep soundly.

Chapter 7: Weekend and Off-Day Adjustments

Balancing Rest and Activity

- **Rest Doesn't Mean Inactivity**: While weekends are great for recharging, staying completely inactive can make you feel sluggish. Instead, find joyful and restorative ways to move your body. Try out activities like a gentle yoga session, nature walks, or even family bike rides. Movement doesn't have to be intense—it's about enjoying your body's natural rhythm. This keeps your energy levels up and prepares you for the week ahead. Weekends can also be a great time to explore new hobbies that keep you active, such as paddle boarding, gardening, or dancing.

- **Social and Emotional Rest**: In addition to physical rest, make time for emotional and social rest. This could involve unplugging from technology, practicing self-care rituals like reading or journaling, or spending time with loved ones. Resting your mind from constant work-related or personal stress helps restore balance, allowing you to approach the new week with a clearer mindset.

- **Prioritize Sleep**: If you haven't gotten enough sleep during the week, weekends are an opportunity to catch up. However, maintaining a regular sleep schedule is important. Avoid sleeping in too much, as this can disrupt your natural sleep cycle and make it harder to wake up on Monday morning. Instead, take short naps or go to bed earlier to allow your body to recover fully.

Meal Preparation for the Week

- **Batch Cooking and Freezing**: Planning and preparing meals in advance helps you avoid unhealthy choices during your busy week. Batch cooking is not only time-efficient, but it also ensures that you always have healthy meals ready to go, reducing stress and saving time during the week. Opt for versatile dishes like soups, curries, casseroles, and roasted vegetables, which can be frozen and reheated easily. Preparing these in large quantities will save you from having to cook every day. You can also pre-portion meals into individual containers, making it easy to grab a balanced meal when you're in a hurry.

- **Smart Grocery Shopping:** Planning meals ahead allows for more efficient grocery shopping. Write a list based on your meal plan and stick to it. This not only helps you avoid impulse buys but also ensures you have all the ingredients on hand for healthy meals. Include a mix of fresh vegetables, lean proteins, whole grains, and healthy fats in your shopping to keep meals balanced. You can even prepare healthy snacks, like chopped veggies or boiled eggs, so they're ready when you need them.

- **Use Your Freezer Wisely**: Make the freezer your best friend! Batch-freeze foods like grains, proteins, and vegetables. You can also freeze individual smoothie packs with fruit, spinach, and other superfoods for a quick, healthy breakfast. By freezing meals in portions, you avoid waste and can easily reheat and enjoy nutrient-dense options on busy days.

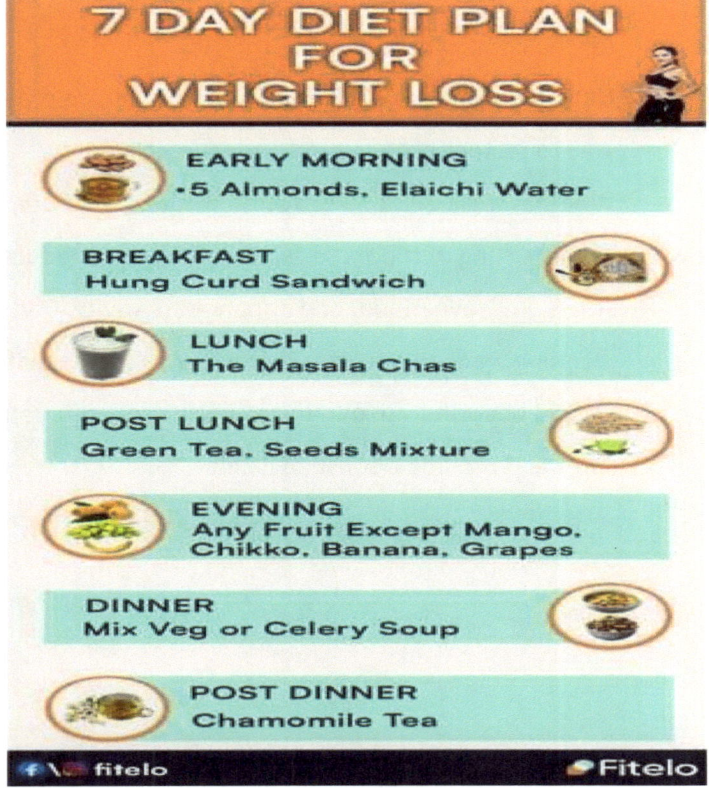

Self-Care and Mental Recharge

- **Mindful Downtime**: Incorporate mindful activities like meditation, journaling, or even creative pursuits such as painting or playing music. This can help you mentally recharge and de-stress from the week. Weekends are an ideal time to reconnect with yourself, reflect on the previous week, and set personal or professional goals for the coming days.

- **Nature and Fresh Air**: Spending time in nature is a great way to restore both mental and physical energy. Whether it's a quiet hike, a stroll through the park, or simply sitting outdoors to read, nature helps reduce stress, improve mood, and enhance creativity. Consider planning weekend outings that allow you to enjoy fresh air and beautiful surroundings, which can uplift your spirit and provide a sense of calm.

Conclusion

Recap of Key Points

☐ **Sustainability is Key**: Living a healthy lifestyle isn't about perfection, but rather building habits you can stick to in the long term. Small, consistent changes add up to big results over time.

Encourage Consistency

☐ **Remind Readers of Their Why**: Staying consistent can be hard, but remembering the reasons for wanting to live healthier (whether for more energy, better focus, or improved mental health) can keep them motivated through tough days.

Final Words on Living a Healthy Lifestyle

☐ **Celebrate Progress**: Each day is an opportunity to make small changes that lead to a healthier life. Celebrate the journey and progress, not just the destination. Recognizing these milestones helps build lasting motivation.